T0144836

# Dr. Earl Mindell's RUSSIAN ENERGY SECRET

## HOW ADAPTOGEN POWER:
- Increases Your Energy, Endurance, and Vitality
- Gives You Deep Immune Support
- Slows the Aging Process

Earl L. Mindell, R.Ph., Ph.D. &
Donald R. Yance, Jr., C.N., M.H.

The information contained in this book is based upon the research and personal and professional experiences of the author. It is not intended as a substitute for consulting with your physician or other health care provider. Any attempt to diagnose and treat an illness should be done under the direction of a health care professional.

The publisher does not advocate the use of any particular health care protocol but believes the information in this book should be available to the public. The publisher and author are not responsible for any adverse effects or consequences resulting from the use of the suggestions, preparations or procedures discussed in this book. Should the reader have any questions concerning the appropriateness of any procedures or preparation mentioned, the author and the publisher strongly suggest consulting a professional health care advisor.

Series Cover Designer: The Great American Art Company
Editor: Susan E. Davis
Typesetter: Gary A. Rosenberg

Basic Health Guides are published by
  Basic Health Publications, Inc.

Copyright © 2001 by Earl Mindell, R.Ph., Ph.D.

ISBN: 978-1-59120-000-0 (Pbk.)
ISBN: 978-1-68162-712-0 (Hardcover)

# Contents

# What Are Adaptogens and What's the Best Way to Use Them?

In 1969 Soviet scientist I.I. Brekhman, Ph.D. reported that the Soviet soldiers who took ginseng extract were able to run a faster in a 3-kilometer race than soldiers who were given a placebo or blank supplement. Dr. Brekhman was the first to call ginseng an adaptogen, which he described as a substance that enables the body to better cope with stress. According to Dr. Brekhman, an adaptogen has the unique ability to normalize body functions. For example, if your blood sugar levels drop too low or if your blood pressure climbs too high, an adaptogen will bring your body back to normal levels. Adaptogens work best with people who are not in poor or peak health but actually somewhere between the two conditions. Since most people fall into this category, supplementing with a liquid adaptogen herbal extract would help their health and feeling of well-being greatly.

The best adaptogenic formula should include one or more flavonoid-rich plants in concentrated liquid form. A mixture of herbs will act in a harmonic way that produces a synergistic effect. This means that the sum of the individual ingredients is much greater than if each one were taken separately.

# The Top 12 Benefits of Adaptogenic Power

1. Increases your energy, endurance and vitality.

2. Enhances your body's own natural defense system, providing deep immune support; increases resistance to a wide range of stresses; reduces the frequency of common infections and speeds recovery.

3. Helps you cope with all areas of stress and protects your body from damage, especially that which is stress induced.

4. Promotes cardiovascular health by strengthening your heart and circulation.

5. Assists in recovery and healing from chronic illness, surgery, chemotherapy and radiation therapy. It can help build bone marrow and restore normal blood levels that had been suppressed.

6. Enhances your brain function, helping preserve neurological function, reducing free radical damage to neurons and improving brain circulation.

7. Aids sleep.

8. Boosts sexual energy by increasing vital essences and circulation.

9. Slows the aging process by providing a potent and diverse antioxidant effect and activating other antioxidant systems in the body. Modulates cellular reduction/oxidation reactions, reduces oxidative stress, neutralizes and prevents free radical damage and promotes more efficient oxygen use. Better oxygen use means less oxidative damage, which translates to better and longer health.

10. Protects the liver and helps restore optimal liver function, preventing damage caused by chemicals in food, the environment and other sources like drugs.

11. Enhances and helps harmonize better overall endocrine function, strengthening hormonal and glandular activity. This includes adrenal, thyroid, pancreas, pineal and thymus function, as well as activities of the reproductive organs.

12. Speeds up trauma recovery, stimulating regeneration and repair by anabolic action.

# Adaptogens:
# New Conceptions,
# Uses and Recent
# Scientific Advances

Though the current model of conventional medicine would have us think otherwise, humans, like plants and all living beings, differ from machines and are not meant to merely function. Humans are meant to create, respond, adapt, heal and love. In today's modern world, stress contributes to at least 70 percent of all illnesses. More than one hundred years ago, the eclectic physician Eli Jones referred to "worriment of the mind" as the number one cause of cancer. Our adaptive capability is critical not only in our ability to resist disease but also in our ability to thrive and be full of zest and zeal.

We live in a progressively fragmented world, and natural medicine is not immune to the tendency to address one type of cancer treatment or one isolated health factor at a time: diet, exercise, chemicals, past lives and so on. In today's fast-paced world, individuals have difficulty paying attention to even one of these disease factors and trying to figure out what's right. For instance, people ask: Should I eat macrobiotic or only raw foods? When one looks at the mainstream American lifestyle, it is a life of frantic time schedules, fast food, sedentary work and chronic high stress. Yet when viewed in the big picture, it's really so mundane, meaningless and often nonhuman.

We need to choose consciously to live in a way that aligns us with our higher principles, based on the harmony between and within our spiritual, environmental and health-oriented self. Chronic stress is at an all-time high; chronic illnesses, including cancer, affect most of the population. Even new "magic silver-bullet cures" cannot heal our polluted environment and bodies.

All aspects of healing are interrelated and are forever in motion. Illness is not something separate from self. As a matter of fact, cancer is very much part of self. If aspects of illness are a combination of our external environment and our internal environment, how can we believe that only outside treatment can be entirely effective? Conventional treatments, however, can play a very important role. Sometimes, on the other hand, they can be a main contributor to disease. Conventional medicine should never replace the traditional healing methods used by all cultures since the beginning of human existence—prayer, music, touch, herbs and healing foods, water and, most of all, love.

Responding to a stimulus can be perceived mostly as the state by which we react to the external environment. How we live, eat, breathe, exercise and rest all contribute to our ability to maintain homeostasis. It's not only a matter of what happens, but how we react to it and how much reserve we have. Over time the accumulation of stress weakens our adaptive capabilities to a point where we fall out of balance. That state of imbalance precedes any manifestation of chronic illness, and the best time to address the person is *before disease sets in.*

Overwhelming evidence has demonstrated that any type of stress has a detrimental effect on the body's ability to maintain optimal levels of important immunological response activities, including the ability of natural killer (NK) cells to destroy viral and cancer cells. A high degree of stress has also been shown to significantly predict a poorer response to interventions aimed at improving NK-cell activity (Kelly). This means that adaptogens are vitally important immune-enhancing agents, particularly effective at assisting in immune response during times of stress.

In conjunction with creating and living a healthy life, one can use herbal adaptogens as important components for enhancing vitality, balance, stress management and the prevention of disease. Herbal adaptogens assist the body because of their ability to normalize homeostasis, optimize metabolism and improve resistance to a variety of adverse factors with few or no side effects. They help us cope with stress not just physiologically, but also mentally and emotionally. They enable us to stay strong and healthy during times when we might otherwise get weak and sick. They also help us resist or delay many of the negative effects of aging by providing us with better physical, mental and sexual energy; for instance, they delay the effects of aging of the eye, skin, heart and all the organ systems. They improve sleep that might otherwise be disrupted by stress. In summary, herbal adaptogens hold great promise for the development and prevention of chronic illness due to their ability to enhance our resistance to a variety of adverse influences.

Prolonged stress leads to suppressed activity of antioxidant systems and immune function, increased lipid peroxidation and increased inflammation. The vast research on adaptogens suggests that these agents possess unique pharmacological properties. They can maintain antioxidant function under normal conditions and can raise our antioxidant abilities under stressful conditions.

Adaptagens are the foundation of any herbal formulation and protocol for anyone with or without cancer. Adaptogens, by themselves, are usually not enough to reverse active cancers, but they should be included in a protocol or formula with other specific herbs in a complementary approach. Adaptogens will enhance the quality and quantity of life. Therefore they are recommended for people who have had active cancer and are now trying to live a healthy and complete life while keeping their cancer dormant.

If we truly believe stress is a main contributing factor to cancer, other chronic illnesses and the aging process and if we truly want to be holistic in our approach to treating causative factors, then adaptogens should be an important aspect of preventing cancer and promoting well-being.

# The Concept of Adaptogens Comes from Russia

Although the term "adaptogen" originated in Russia, the practice of using herbs on a daily basis to prevent disease, to slow down the aging process, to enhance health and well-being and to increase one's ability to cope with stress has been used in Chinese medicine for thousands of years. Using such herbs as ginseng provided great endurance and strength needed to ensure survival in harsh conditions. The wisdom inherent in Chinese medicine was passed down from generation to generation.

Many of the classic adaptogens, including *Eleutherococcus senticosus*, *Panax pseudoginseng*, *Panax quinquefolium* and *Oplopanax horridum*, are all members of the Araliaceae family.

In the 1950s Russian scientists began to study these plants individually, and over the past 40 years more than 2,000 scientific studies have been done on adaptogens. Unfortunately, the current Western scientific model of assessing the beneficial effects of herbs, or anything at all, is not adequate to truly assess the benefits adaptogens provide for all people wanting to have optimum health. Modern science does provide an invaluable point of view, but it must be seen as simply that—a point of view. As noted naturopath Deborah Frances has noted: "In a world which has granted supremacy to a scientific point of view, objectivity reigns and subjectivity is often totally rejected. Double blind studies are allowed to negate personal experiences, and only that which can be physically measured and quantified is accepted as real. Such a one-sided approach severely hampers our ability to be whole, not only in our approach to medicine, but in our lives in general."

The hypothesis about the state of enhanced general resistance (SEGR) was developed in Russia in 1959 by leading pharmacologist and professor N. V. Lazarev and remains crucial for understanding the action of adaptogens. In the 1950s and 1960s much testing with *Eleutherococcus senticosus,* also known as Siberian ginseng, was conducted in Russia on factory workers, truck drivers, sailors on long voyages, military personnel, athletes and cosmonauts (Russian astronauts). The research showed that the administration of Eleutherococcus increased energy, stamina and the capacity to carry out demanding activities while enhancing the ability to handle all types of stressors.

The Russian government realized that this new class of natural substances, most notably Eleutherococcus, could give Russians an advantage in sports, space and the military. Because of this, the government strongly supported scientific research into adaptogens, and more than 2,000 scientific papers (mostly Russian) attest to the effectiveness of Eleutherococcus. (Prior to studying Eleutherococcus, the Russians had been studying *Panax ginseng.* The investigators found Eleutherococcus to be better tolerated by a wide range of people, easier to find or grow and more cost-effective than *Panax ginseng.*)

Eleutherococcus has been shown to be highly effective in improving our ability to respond to adverse conditions. It can help with temperature extremes, immobilization (for example, after surgery or on long airplane flights), cancer therapies, X-rays, the effects of high-dose hormone therapies (insulin, epinephrine, steroids) and jet lag. It also has a preventive effect on the growth of biological pathogens and can improve both mental and physical work capacity.

## PHASES OF ADAPTOGENS' PROTECTIVE ACTION

Adaptogens provide protection for the body during the daily grind and under harmful conditions:

When adaptogens are used under normal conditions, they:

1. Increase work capacity.

2. Activate the organism's systems.

3. Stimulate the defense systems.

When adaptogens are used under stressful (harmful) conditions, they:

1. Activate the organism's endocrine (hormone) and homeostatic systems.

2. Protect from damage (especially stress-induced damage) through anti-catabolic action.

3. Stimulate regeneration and repair through anabolic/anticatabolic action.

Herbalists apply an energetic understanding of all plant medicines including adaptogens. We understand and use the most appropriate herbal adaptogen(s) for the specific constitutional make-up of the individual. Traditional herbal medicines are used for the treatment of stress-induced nervous system exhaustion and fatigue, insomnia, weakness, depression, forgetfulness, vision problems, diarrhea and chemical toxicity. Schizandra seed extract, for example, is a potent antioxidant that has demonstrated its superiority to vitamin antioxidants against selective oxygen species (SOS), also called free radicals. In addition, various ethanol-soluble lignans found in the seed extract have powerful liver-protective properties against a variety of chemical toxins. Besides hepatitis and other liver ailments, Schizandra is also helpful in healing certain types of intestinal infections, including chronic gastritis. Russian studies also indicate that Schizandra improves vision, particularly in adjusting to darkness.

# The Hot 16 Adaptogens

**S**tudies show that the following 16 adaptogens have the most decisive effects on the body's overall well-being.

## 1. SIBERIAN GINSENG (*ELEUTHEROCOCCUS SENTICOSUS*)

Many consider Siberian ginseng, often called Eleutherococcus or simply Eleuthero, the "king" of all adaptogens. It has been shown to be highly effective in improving adaptive capability to such adverse conditions as temperature extremes, immobilization, recovery from injury and from drug intoxication, X-rays, jet 1ag and during the administration of high-dosage hormone therapies (insulin, epinephrine, steroids). In addition, it provides a useful adjunct to cancer therapies and has a preventive effect against the growth of biological pathogens. While also promoting both mental and physical work capacity, this herb increases both mental and physical work capacity, normalizes blood pressure and immune activity and reduces fatigue, stress, depression and atherosclerosis. It also balances the endocrine system and promotes vitality.

Soviet researchers conducted the preponderance of clinical trials of Siberian ginseng that proved its antistress effects on humans, and most have not been published in English language journals. The accumulation of data from Soviet studies indicates that the ingestion of Siberian ginseng extract by humans increases their ability to accommodate to adverse physical conditions, improve mental performance and enhance the quality of work under stressful conditions.

Over 35 compounds have been identified from the roots of Siberian ginseng. One group of compounds, the eleutherosides, has been shown to be primarily responsible for the plant's adaptogenic activity. In addition, according to Wanger and Proksch, two polysaccharides in the root display the immunopotentiating activity (Kelly and Foster).

## 2. AMERICAN AND KOREAN GINSENG (*PANAX QUINQUEFOLIUM/GINSENG*)

Ginseng has been used as a traditional medicine in Asian countries for more than 5,000 years, and more than 500 scientific papers have been published on ginseng throughout the world. There are several types of ginseng, including Chinese and Korean (*Panax ginseng*), which can be either white or red, and American (*Panax quinquefolium*). American ginseng, highly revered throughout Asia, is a bit more cooling than the other types, making it better for people with a fast metabolic rate who tend to "run a bit hot." It is considered a lung tonic in traditional Chinese medicine. The name "Panax" is derived from the Greek *pan,* meaning "all," and *akos,* meaning "remedy," clearly reflecting the root's reputation as a panacea or cure-all.

In China and Korea, ginseng is taken as both a medicine and a power food and is most often classified as an adaptogen. Ginseng is most noted for its antifatigue and antiaging effects. This has been attributed to a group of compounds in ginseng called "ginsenosides." Saponins, yet another group of compounds, have been shown to inhibit the proliferation of tumors induced by various chemicals and have demonstrated some overall antitumor activity. Ginseng has been shown to enhance the overall activity of the immune system, including antibody response, NK-cell activity, interferon production and the proliferate and phacocytic (pathogen-engulfing) ability of the immune system (Huang).

Ginseng extract can potentiate the activity of cytotoxic drugs and radiation therapy. Ginseng also possesses direct anticancer effects involving a vast array of mechanisms, including DNA repair, immune system enhancement and endocrine system enhancement. Ginseng also promotes antimutagenic and antioxidant activity and causes the induction of differentiation in cancer cells (Mills and Bone).

Dr. T. Hisayama and his coworkers in their paper "Clinical experience in the treatment of advanced cancer with ginsenosides" found that ginsenoside administration provides a restorative effect on leukocyte counts and the hemoglobin level of cancer patients exposed to large doses of radiation. Patients recovered from anemia, leukopenia and lymphopenia (Boik, pp. 307–309).

## Stress Management, Exercise and Work Efficiency

Ginseng appears to work on the hypothalamus and has a sparing effect on the adrenal cortex, mediated through stimulation of the anterior pituitary gland and release of ACTH (Adrenal Cortico Tropic Hormone). Response to stress is quicker and more efficient, and feedback control is more effective so that when stress decreases, glucocorticoid levels fall more rapidly to normal (Fulder).

Numerous studies have demonstrated the effects of ginseng on neuropsychological and physical adaptation to external environmental changes and various stresses. Ginseng has been shown to be beneficial in maintaining normal physiological functions for a longer period than in the case of a control group (Duke). Its normalizing properties help regulate all imbalances caused by stress, and for this reason ginseng is considered a restorative. When the body conditions are normalized, it enhances the defense mechanism in a state of impaired physical and neuropsychological functioning (Duke). All this is attributed to ginseng's adaptogenic properties.

In 1951 Dr. Chernenikh of the USSR Academy of Science performed an experiment involving four groups of workers to determine whether ginseng had an effect on work efficiency. He administered wild ginseng extract to the first group after one hour's work, cultivated Korean ginseng extract to the second group, glucose to the third group and alcohol to the last group. Then he compared the accuracy of the work of the four groups before and after the administration. He found that mistakes made by the alcohol-fed group increased 46 percent and those by the glucose-fed group increased by 16 percent, but the group given Korean ginseng made fewer mistakes and the wild ginseng group made the least (Duke).

In 1951 in the USSR Professor Petkov established that daily doses of ginseng preparations over 15 to 45 days increase physical endurance and mental capacity for work as well as industrial activity (Duke). The increase in work efficiency was noted not only during the experiment itself but also for a stated period of time (a month and a half) after the experiment. Professors Petkov and Brekhman remarked in their report to the USSR Academy of Science that there is a world of difference between ginseng and other stimulants such as caffeine or amphetamine (Duke). For example:

- Ginseng is not an excitant. It does not cause feelings of over excitation, emotional disturbance or agitation.

- Ginseng has a sedative component. Unlike with other stimulants, one has no difficulty sleeping after taking it.

- Ginseng acts in a stabilizing fashion. The more tired one is, the more noticeable the action.

- Ginseng causes an increase in health, appetite and mental condition, especially if taken over an extended period. The other stimulants cause more ill health the longer they are taken.

- Ginseng is much safer. It assists in combating stress, while the other stimulants can actually cause stress (Huang).

The herbalist understands that herbs work not just because of their active ingredients but through the total of their combined effects. Extraction of only the active component, which is how most drugs are created today, is not only unnecessary but may even be harmful. "Ginseng is one of the few herbs for which there is clear scientific evidence that there are more medicinal powers in the entire plant than in any of the chemicals so far isolated from it," explained Dr. Stephen Fulder in his book, *The Root of Being: Ginseng and the Pharmacology of Harmony.*

## 3. PANTOCRENE (EXTRACTED FROM THE VELVET OF THE SIBERIAN DEER ANTLER)

Pantocrene is a purified extract taken from the velvet antler of the young Siberian deer (*Cornu cervi parvum*). Classified as a kidney tonic, which fortifies yang, pantocrene is a general tonic that increases work capacity; improves sleep, strength and appetite; decreases the rate of muscle fatigue; and possesses anticatabolic action. It increases physical and sexual energy and also improves clarity of the mind.

### Traditional Uses

- Traditionally pantocrene is used to treat fatigue, impotence, cold extremities, lightheadedness, tinnitus, clear and copious urination, and soreness and lack of strength in the lower back and knees.

- It is also used to strengthen bones and treat anemia, insufficient growth and learning disorders, including mental retardation.

## Modern Uses

- Nowadays pantocrene is used to treat cardiovascular problems, including to increase cardiac output in weak and aged hearts. It also regulates hearts with arrhythmias and improves circulation and blood flow, particularly in individuals with low blood pressure.

- Pantocrene has a general strengthening effect. In animal studies pantocrene increases oxygen uptake of the brain, liver and kidneys, and increases body weight.

- Pantocrene has hematological effects. When red and white blood cells are suppressed, pantocrene increases their production.

- Pantocrene has an immunological effect. When it is given to animals that have been sensitized to a particular substance, pantocrene inhibits a reaction when they are reexposed to that substance. Thus pantocrene is seen to have an anti-allergenic effect.

- Pantocrene promotes wound healing. It helps the granulation of long-standing ulcers and wounds as well as healing bone fractures.

## 4. ARCTIC ROOT (*RHODIOLA ROSEA*)

Based on many years of Russian research, the root of *Rhodiola rosea,* whose common name is "Arctic root," has been shown to rival Eleutherococcus as an important adaptogen. The active constituents in Rhodiola are believed to be two glycosides referred to as "rosavidin," also called "rosavin" and "salidroside." Rhodiloa is well suited for people with adrenal excess who are prone to elevations of blood pressure or blood lipids and who tire easily and have poor stamina and endurance.

Many conditions respond more favorably to Rhodiola extract than other adaptogens like *Panax ginseng,* although we believe that taking a combination of adaptogens offers the most benefit. Rhodiola is superior to ginseng during acute stress because it prevents stress-induced disruptions in function and performance. Rhodiola administrations have been shown to increase serotonin and decrease the enzyme responsible for monoamine degradation, monoamine oxidase and catechol-O-methyltransferase (Stancheva and Mosharrof). Russian research has shown that Rhodiola is also helpful in conditions of depression and schizophrenia and in stress-related damage to cardiovascular tissue.

Much of the research on Rhodiola extract has focused on its ability to assist the body at times of stress, particularly cardiac stress, acting in part to prevent stress-induced catecholamine activity in cardiac tissue and reduce adrenaline-induced arrhythmias in animals. Rhodiola, along with Reishi mushrooms and hawthorn, are excellent adaptogens for people at high risk for cardiovascular disease. Rhodiola extract also protects against altitude sickness, minimizing cardiopulmonary dysfunction.

In addition to Rhodiola's protective effects on the nervous and endocrine system, it possesses anticarcinogenic, antimetastatic and antimutagenic activity. In oncology, the use of adaptogenic plants, including Rhodiola, Eleutherococcus, Schizandra and *Rhaponticum carthamoides,* has been shown to consistently improve results (Zhou and Liu). There is enough evidence based on years of research to conclude that adaptogenic plants, including Rhodiola, along with other adaptogens when used regularly, can effectively prevent the development and reoccurrence of cancer, suppress metastases and decrease the adverse side effects of conventional cytotoxic therapies. In animal experiments, adding Rhodiola extract to a protocol with Adriamycin resulted in an improved inhibition of tumor dissemination (compared to Adriamycin alone), and the combined protocol prevented liver toxicity (Odintsev).

Rhodiola extract has also been shown to enhance the antitumor effects of the hemotherapeutic drug cyclophosphamide (Cytoxin), while at the same time assisting in the regenerative process of the immune system (Yaremenko and Pashinski). Rhodiola has been shown to shorten the recovery time of suppressed white blood cells following chemotherapy or radiation treatment (Yaremenko and Pashinski).

## 5. SCHIZANDRA (SEED AND FRUIT) OR MAGNOLIA VINE (*SCHIZANDRA CHINENSIS*)

Schizandra, which means "five flavor fruit," has a long history as a valuable tonic—an adaptogen with a diverse range of indications for use. Schizandra has a stimulating effect on the central nervous system without being excitatory and enhances both mental and physical capabilities. Schizandra is widely used for the treatment of stress-induced nervous system exhaustion and fatigue, insomnia, weakness, depression, forgetfulness, diarrhea and chemical toxicity. It is also used for regulating gastric secretions to balance pH levels and for a variety of liver ailments, including both viral and chemically induced hepatitis. Schizandra is especially effective at lowering serum transaminase levels. It is without a doubt one of herbalists' favorite herbs, and we use it as a general tonic as well as an aid in detoxification. It is especially helpful in helping rid the body of chemical toxins, including those introduced by chemotherapy and radiation therapy (Sinclair).

As an anxioxidant Schizandra has demonstrated its superiority to vitamin antioxidants against oxygen-free radicals. Various ethanol-soluble lignans in the seed extract have been shown to exert strong liver-protective actions against an array of chemical toxins. Besides helping to cure hepatitis and other liver ailments, Schizandra helps heal certain types of intestinal infections, including chronic gastritis. Soviet studies also indicate that Schizandra plays a role in improving vision, notably helping the eye adjust to darkness (Wahlstrom).

Most of the research on Schizandra as an adaptogen has been done on the seed extract rather than on the fruit. Yet the encapsulated Schizandra fruit or fruit extracts are sold widely in the United States. Although the fruit is a good medicine, possessing astringent properties and acting as a kidney-lung tonic as well as an adaptogen, it is not nearly as potent as the seed. The best Schizandra is made only from the seed.

Schizandra's effects include:

1. Antitoxic and antioxidant activity against many chemical toxicities. Protects DNA from damage (most notably carbon tetrachloride, which is activated in the body into a potent liver toxin called peroxyl trichloromethyl that induces rapid lipid peroxidation).

2. Induction of liver-detoxifying enzymes, Phase I (cytochrome P450) and Phase II (glutathioneS-transferase).

3. Stimulation of the biosynthesis of protein and liver glycogen.

4. Calming of the mind and heart, particularly when blood or yin deficiency is present. It also increases energy and stamina and improves sleep.

5. Improvement of eyesight, hearing and mental acuity, especially when impaired due to liver and kidney deficiency.

6. Adaptogen activity: balancing, normalizing and overall strengthening of the entire body.

## 6. ASHWAGANDHA ROOT (*WITHANIA SOMNIFERA*)

Ashwagandha is one of the most revered plants in Ayurvedic medicine. This herb grows throughout the southern part of India. It is classified as a tonic-adaptogen and is often referred to as the "Indian ginseng," although not related botanically to ginseng.

### Traditional Uses

Ashwagandha is used to treat asthma, bronchitis, psoriasis, arthritis, insomnia, nervous exhaustion, and dementia, and to promote conception. Ashwagandha has long been used as an aphrodisiac in Ayurvedic medicine, and it is used as a restorative for those weakened by stress or long illness.

### Modern Uses

Ashwagandha is used to promote growth, anti-anemic and anti-aging activity; to improve stamina and athletic performance; to offset the side effects of cancer drug and radiation; to cure impotence due to exhaustion; and as a general tonic to prevent disease and reduce the effects of stress.

Active constituents within the root include alkaloids (isopelietierine and snaferine), steroidal lacrones (withanolides, withaferins), saponins (including sitoindoside VII, VIII) and the mineral iron.

When Ashwagandha is compared with *Panax ginseng,* it has demonstrated a similar potency to Panax as an adaptogenic tonic and to its anabolic effects (Grandhi).

### Use in Cancer Therapy

• Ashwagandha has been shown to significantly increase white blood cell and neutrophil counts before and after treatment with the chemotherapeutic drug cyclophosphamide (Ganasoundari).

• Ashwagandha has recently been shown to have antitumor and radiosensitizing effects in experimental tumors in vivo, without any systemic toxicity. It is recommended during and after radiation therapy (Devi).

## 7. OATS (STRAW, GRAIN AND FRESH MILKY UNRIPE SEED) (*AVENA SATIVA*)

The fresh extract made from the milky seed of oats (*Avena sativa*) strengthens and nourishes the nervous system. It is used for neurasthenia (nervous exhaustion, "that stressed-out feeling"), anxiety, impaired sleep patterns, weakness and poor libido, and as a tonic for those who are burning the candle at both ends. Milky oats are a nutritive tonic, rich in minerals, in particular calcium and magnesium, which are important nutrients for the nervous system.

A classic nervine tonic, oats both builds energy and reduces stress. It also raises the mood and is useful in combating addictions to such substances as tobacco, cannabis and opium. It is the best remedy for feeding the nervous system, and it helps restore vital energy and recovery from illness and/or prolonged times of stress. Although not always listed as a classic adaptogen, it is considered to be one by many herbalists. For instance, Dr. Finley Ellingwood says, "Avena is a remedy of great utility in loss of nerve power and in muscular feebleness from lack of nerve force."

The constitutents of *Avena sativa* include proteins, prolamines known as avenins, C-Glycosyl flavones, Avenacosides known as spirostanol glycosides, calcium, magnesium and vitamin E.

## *MEDICINAL MUSHROOMS*

Medicinal mushrooms have immunomodulating activities and have been used as tonics in traditional Chinese medicine (TCM). They are now used in cancer treatments to counteract the toxic effects of chemotherapy and radiation therapy. Mushrooms used in cancer therapies are generally processed into liquid or powdered form in order to obtain the necessary potency. For example, about 15 pounds of Reishi mushrooms are required to produce one pound of the powdered concentrate. Medicinal mushrooms' most significant contribution to the healing process is the enhancement and stimulation of the body's own immune system—a very important factor in diseases like cancer and HIV infection (AIDS).

## 8. REISHI MUSHROOM (*GANODERMA LUCIDUM*)

Reishi mushroom (*Ganoderma lucidum*) is traditionally used in Chinese medicine for asthenia-type syndromes, which are characterized by a deficiency of vital energy and lower body functions. In Chinese medicine, the Reishi is called "Ling Zhi," which means "spirit plant," and is known to increase longevity. Reishi's overall effects could be described as regulatory and beneficial to the restoration of homeostasis. Its effect on the immune system is total enhancement of functioning, including an increase in white blood cell count, platelets, hemoglobin and various tumor-fighting cells. Reishi also improves both energy and sleep. Traditionally Reishi is used in the treatment of hyperlipemia, chronic bronchitis, hepatitis and leukopenia.

The main activities of Reishi include the following:

- Oxygen-free radical scavenger.
- Hypolipidemic (cholesterol lowering).
- Antiatherosclerotic (inhibits platelet aggregation).
- Cardiovascular regulating.
- Immunomodulator.
- Hepatoprotective.
- Hypoglycemic (lowers blood sugar).
- Stress-reducing effect.
- Preventing and combating altitude sickness.
- Antisenescence (retards the aging process).

Being a true adaptogen, Reishi enhances the healthy, normal functions of the body but also works therapeutically to address imbalances. Reishi is used for conservation and promotion of good health, but it is also good for age-related illnesses (such as hypertension), coronary heart disease and cancer (Huang, pp. 118–20). Reishi is the perfect remedy for the typical American suffering from constant stress. This type of individual has repressed vital force and is likely to be both deficient (depleted) and toxic. When a person in such a state develops cancer and is then faced with the toxicities of chemotherapy, the situation calls for Reishi.

One study showed that Reishi strongly inhibited the growth of sarcoma-180, with an inhibition rate of 95.6 to 98.6 percent at an intraperitoneal dosage of 20 mg/kg for 10 days in mice (Lien and Li). Another study demonstrated that Reishi polysaccharides significantly inhibited the proliferation of JTC-26 tumor cells, a human cancer cell strain (Zhou and Liu). Ganoderic acids U-Z, which are six types of cytotoxic triterpenes found in Reishi, showed significant cytotoxicity on hepatoma cells grown in vitro (Cheng).

Due to its stimulating effects on bone marrow, Reishi can protect the body during radiation and chemotherapy. Clinical studies have shown Reishi to be effective in the treatment of leukopenia induced by radiation, chemical agents or other factors. Reishi also improved symptoms of weakness, dizziness, sleeplessness and elevated or suppressed blood counts.

Ganoderma polysaccharides promote the production of IL-2 and markedly enhance the cytotoxicity of T-lymphocytes. The extract also has the effect of delaying hypersensitivity; it modulates immune response and reduces allergic or autoimmune reactions (Ho; Jianzhe).

## 9. CORDYCEPS (*CORDYCEPS SINENSIS*)

Cordyceps is found in the highlands of China, Nepal and Tibet at elevations above 10,000 feet. In China it is called "winter worm, summer grass and the caterpillar mushroom." Cordyceps is a form of fungus that grows on the larvae of the caterpillar *Hepialus comoricanus oberthuer.* Considered one of the most valuable medicinal herbs used traditionally in China, it equals ginseng as a restorative tonic. Active constituents of Cordyceps include polysaccharides, cordycepin, sterols, adenosine and cordycepic acid. Between 25 and 32 percent of the herb consists of crude protein, cordycepin 3-decoxyadenosine and d-mannitol

According to Li Chih Shen, the great sixteenth-century herbalist, Cordyceps can invigorate and tone the entire body. It is particularly useful as a tonic that builds vitality during recovery from stress, illness or physical challenges. Cordyceps, traditionally cooked in soups like many of the other medicinal mushrooms, builds the bone marrow and is classified in traditional Chinese medicine as a kidney and lung tonic. Although Cordyceps tonifies both yin and yang, it predominately tonifies yang and is used to treat impotence and a sore, weak lower back (deficient kidney yang). It is considered a safe herb to use long term.

Cordyceps is particularly protective of the kidneys and is an effective treatment for renal disease. The herb exhibits protective effects against aminoglycoside nephrotoxicity in geriatric patients and protects against cyclosporine A-induced nephrotoxicity in rats. Cordyceps has been shown to increase creatinine clearance, increase hemoglobin and stimulation of reticulocytes in the blood count and also decrease blood urea nitrogen (BUN). It is antiasthmatic, assists smooth muscle relaxation and can potentiate the effects of epinephrine (Huang).

The main activities of Cordyceps include the following:

- Oxygen-free radical scavenger.

- Antisenescent (retards the aging process).

- Endocrine modulator.

- Hypolipidemic (cholesterol lowering).

- Antiatherosclerotic.

- Immunomodulator.

- Restorer of sexual function and replenisher of sperm.

- Renal, hepatic, respiratory, nervous system and cardiovascular tonic.

- Stress reducer.

- Promoter of endurance, vigor and energy; enhanced training and perfomance in athletic competition

Cordyceps attracted public attention in 1993 when a group of Chinese runners broke nine world records in the World Outdoor Track and Field Championships in Germany. Afterward the coach partially attributed those results to the athletes' use of a Cordycep-based tonic (Hobbs).

Cordyceps exhibits an immunopotentiating effect in treating cancer and immunodeficient patients. It increases IL-2, interferon, NK cells, and TNF production. A warm-water extract prepared from dried *Cordyceps sinensis* was tested for antitumor activity in vivo in mice given a carcinogen and then exposed to whole body radiation. After 60 days, eight of the ten mice given Cordyceps extract were still alive while none of the control group survived (Zhou and Lin).

Although Cordycepin and the cordycep-polysaccharides are believed to be the active immunomodulatory compounds, an extract of

Cordyceps with the polysaccharides removed showed effective cancer inhibitory effects (Kuo). The ethanol extract of Cordyceps has been shown to be a potent immune-enhancing agent as well as an inhibitor of several cancer cell lines. These include B16 melanoma, K562, Vero, Wish, Calu-1, Rajii and HA22T/VGH tumor cell lines. A clinical trial on 36 patients with advanced cancer showed that this herb can restore cellular immunological functions and improve the quality of their life significantly (Zhou and Lin).

## 10. LICORICE (*GLYCYRRHIZA GLABRA*)

Licorice possesses antiviral activity. It is an anti-inflammatory, antitumor and antiulcer herb, and it increases the production of interferon and NK-cell activity. Licorice inhibits expression of the Epstein Barr virus and the development of certain cancers as well as chronic fatigue syndrome and herpes. It also possesses liver-protective and antiallergenic activity and protects the thymus and adrenal gland from the stress hormone cortisone. Triferpenes, mainly glycyrrhizin, can block tumor-promoting agents. A recent study done in Japan demonstrated that glycyrrhizin could inhibit liver cancer caused by hepatitis (Arase).

### Traditional Uses

Licorice has been used for thousands of years throughout the world for a variety of health conditions. This includes irritation to mucous membranes of the urinary, respiratory and digestive tracts, leading to such ailments as bronchitis, coughs and stomach ulcers. Licorice also reduces adrenal fatigue. In Chinese medicine, licorice was classified as a spleen tonic that removes heat and moistens the mucous membranes. It moderates and harmonizes the characteristics of other plants.

Chinese medical texts describe licorice as an agent to "improve the tone of the digestive system" and replenish vitality, remove heat and toxins, moisten the lungs and arrest coughing and relieve pain and spasm. Licorice increases overall vitality. It is also considered a synergist and used in many classic formulas as a supporting and harmonizing agent (Huang).

The flavonoids and isoflavonoids in licorice can regulate hormones, and the polysaccharide fraction has immunostimulating activity. Licorice modulates IL-2 production and the proliferation of murine thymocytes in response to the anti-CD-3 monoclonal antibody. The herb activates T-cells in the liver. Licorice is a potent antitoxin, lowering the toxicity of many poisons, including strychnine, histamine, arsenate, snake venom, diphtheria, tetanus and others.

Licorice affects adrenal function by increasing the production of cortisol and aiding the conversion of cortisol to cortisone on demand. Licorice also increases the production of DHEA and aldosterone, both important hormones made by the adrenal glands. Increased cortisol produces anti-inflammatory actions and may inhibit the growth of leukemia and lymphoma cells by affecting glucocorticoid receptor sites on their plasma membranes.

## FLAVONOID-RICH PLANTS AS ADAPTOGENS

Flavonoids are a group of compounds found extensively in the plant kingdom. Flavonoid molecules have a distinctive structure consisting of multiple phenolic rings that are usually substituted by hydroxyl groups.

We consider certain flavonoid-rich plants to be adaptogens because they act in such broad beneficial and diverse ways. The flavonoid-rich plants most often prescribed include elderberry (*Sambuccua canadensis nigra*), the leaf, flower and berry of bilberry or blueberry (*Vaccinium myrtillus*); the leaf, flower and berry of hawthorn (*Crataegus oxyacantha*); the skin and seed of the red and/or purple grape (*Vitis vinifera*); and the common cranberry (*Vaccinium oxycoccos*). We recommend that everyone consume at least one source of these important plant-based, flavonoid-rich adaptogens regularly, whether as food or as an herbal supplement.

One way to determine which flavonoid-rich berry should be ingested as a supplement in a concentrated form for a particular individual is based on body systems. Each supplement has a specific affinity for an area of the body: hawthorn, the heart and cardiovascular system; bilberry, the eye; cranberry, the urinary tract; elderberry, the immune system; and grape, the lymph and liver. Grape juice has been used throughout Europe as a nutritive adaptogenic tonic both for cleansing and for strengthening the body.

## 11. ELDERBERRY (*SAMBUCCUA CANADENSIS NIGRA*)

In 400 B.C. Hippocrates referred to the elder tree as his "medicine chest." Similar to hawthorn berries and blueberries, the elderberry is a concentrated source of the purple-blue pigment flavonoids, referred to as anthocyanidins, that benefit the health in a variety of ways. Flavonoids occur in most plant species and account for a significant percentage of the chemical constituents found in certain plants. Flavonoids act as potent inhibitors of oxidative damage through their ability to scavenge a wide range of free radicals, including hydroxyl, superoxide anions and lipid peroxy radicals. Flavonoids have also been shown to have potent anti-inflammatory, antimutagenic, antiviral, antibacterial, antineoplastic, antithrombotic and vasodilatory activity. Since oxidative damage is implicated in most or all chronic illnesses, the diet should include flavonoid-rich plants and a flavonoid extract should be added to a supplement regimen.

Recent studies of elderberry extract have shown that it possesses an array of health benefits, including:

1. Potent free-radical scavenging ability, reducing oxidative stress (antioxidant) and providing cellular protection.

2. Nonspecific immune enhancement, boosting cytokine production. A unique protein found in elderberry acts as a messenger regulating immune response.

3. Antiviral activity, which allows elderberry to act as a potent viral inhibitor. Its anti-influenza ability is much researched in both Israel and Switzerland. Elderberry has also been shown to inhibit the herpes virus and the HIV virus in cell culture. Elderberry can be taken as a tonic to inhibit colds and the flu.

4. Cardiovascular protection, reducing LDL cholesterol and atherosclerosis. The anthocyanidins present in elderberries protect vascular epithelial cells against oxidative insult, preventing vascular disease.

5. Stress reduction, with Austrian research showing that elderberry possesses a remarkable stress-reducing and adaptogenic ability. In one study, elderberry shortened recovery time from physical exertion, and in another study conducted by the U.S. Air Force, elderberry extract reduced the stress load endured by pilots (Porter).

6. Collagen-stabilizing action. This makes elderberry useful for healing connective tissue swelling, both acute and chronic. This includes hemorrhoids, sprains, arthritis and varicose veins.

## 12. HAWTHORN (LEAVES, BLOSSOMS AND BERRIES) (*CRATAEGUS OXYACANTHA*)

The leaves, blossoms and berries of hawthorn all contain an abundant amount of active compounds. The most important components are flavonoids, some of which include anthocyanidins and proanthocyanidins, triterpenes and aromatic dioxides. Hawthorn is the cardiac-tonic plant medicine widely prescribed by Western herbalists for the heart and vascular system. The effects of hawthorn are slow but steady.

Specific indications and main uses of hawthorn are for:

- Hypertension: works best in arterial type hypertension. Because it's slow acting, hawthorn needs to be taken for several months before a noticeable drop in blood pressure occurs.

- Mild cases of coronary insufficiency, especially due to age.

- Sensitivity to cardiac glycosides.

- Myocarditis, which is inflammation of the heart following contagious disease such as rheumatic fever (damaged heart from endomyocarditis or pericarditis).

- Right-lobe failure.

- Damage to coronary arteries.

- Angina pectoris: gives relief for cramplike pain and may, after time, bring permanent relief from pain (combine with magnesium potassium orotate and bromelain).

- Valvular deficiency.

- General tonic for anyone who has had a heart attack and/or wants to prevent one. Improves coronary blood flow and restores myocardial reserve.

- Gentle nervine: useful when there is mild heart disease and with nervousness, in which case it can be combined with oats, motherwort, cactus, lemon balm, Reishi and Chinese sage (dan shen or *Salvia miltiorrhiza*).

- Tachycardia (rapid heart rate) and other functional cardiac disturbances; can be combined with digitalis or beta-blockers *only under proper supervision.* We often use hawthorn and other herbs either to help get someone off these medications or to enable them to use a reduced dosage while still maintaining the desired effects of the medication.

- Connective tissue swelling, both acute and chronic. Due to hawthorn's collagen-stabilizing action, it is useful for healing such conditions as hemorrhoids, sprains, arthritis and varicose veins.

- Fat loss: Hawthorn can contribute to fat loss because it increases the body's ability to use fatty acids for energy. In traditional Chinese medicine (TCM), hawthorn is used to treat obesity. Also in TCM, hawthorn is used to treat digestive weakness, the symptoms of which include bloating, dyspepsia and diarrhea.

- Symptoms of coronary heart disease: A hawthorn extract has been shown in clinical trials to relieve such symptoms, including stress tolerance, more effectively than the ACE inhibitor captopril (Donald Brown's Review).

## 13. GRAPE SEED AND SKIN EXTRACT (*VITIS VINIFERA*)

Grape seed extract is a rich source of anthocyanidins, proanthocyanidins and oligomer proanthocyanidins, which are flavonoids that give many fruits, in particular berries, their dark purple and blue color. These flavonoids' free-radical-scavenging effects are 20 to 50 times greater than that of vitamin C or E. These flavonoids also reinforce the natural cross-linking of collagen that forms the matrix of connective tissue, a very important function during any postsurgical healing. They are anti-inflammatory because they prevent the release and synthesis of compounds that promote inflammation such as histamines, serine proteases and prostaglandins. Such characteristics make grape seed extract useful as an anti-inflammatory in adjunctive nutritional support with primary treatment of hemorrhoids, swollen joints, athletic injuries, cancer inhibition and postsurgical edema and lymphoma. The extract is also helpful as a cardiovascular tonic and for its general antiaging ability.

Within the grape skin is the polyphenolic compound called resveratrol, which is one of the strongest natural cyclooxygenase-2 (COX-2) inhibitors known. It possesses chemopreventive properties and functions as a plant-defense molecule. Resveratrol inhibits cancer by many mechanisms, including anti-inflammatory activity, antioxidant action and induction of phase II detoxifying enzymes in the liver.

COX-2 appears to be overexpressed in most if not all cancers and correlates very tightly with carcinogenesis in a number of target organs (almost every target organ we've seen so far): cancer of the head and neck, bladder, colon, pancreas, breast and prostate. Dr. Ernest Hawk of the National Cancer Institute in Bethesda, Maryland, said that it may be possible to intervene at every stage—from pre-invasive lesions to advanced cancers—in a broad range of organs. "And I note," added Dr. Hawk, "that there is additional work suggesting that overexpression of COX-2 exists among almost every other tumor, in both animal models as well as [in] human settings" (Dannenberg; Harris).

## 14. GREEN TEA (*CAMELLIA SINENSIS*)

Green tea (*Camellia sinensis*), which has been consumed on a daily basis throughout Asia for hundreds of years, generally supports overall health and stamina and reduces fatigue. It shows numerous health-promoting biological activities from cancer inhibition, antioxidant and cardiovascular protection, all the way to ergogenic effects. Green tea also has specific health benefits for the pancreas by improving insulin utilization, and it helps strengthen connective tissue. In addition to containing a small amount of caffeine—about 14 percent, which is significantly less than is found in coffee—green tea's active compounds are a group of polyphenols called catechins.

Green tea phenolic and polyphenolic compounds, which include Epigallocatechin-3-gallate (EGCG), the most abundant phenolic-flavonoid compound found in green tea, are potent antioxidants and anticancer agents. EGCG's ability to inhibit cancer is multifunctional and includes antioxidant, antiallergenic, antiviral, adaptogen qualities and the capacity to activate certain detoxifying systems. Green tea gives us broad protection against four major categories of carcinogens:

1. Indirect chemical carcinogens (such as benzopyrene in diesel fuel).

2. Direct chemical carcinogens (such as nitrates in processed meats).

3. Physical carcinogens (such as ultraviolet [UV] light).

4. Tumor promoters (such as DDT).

Green tea inhibits the formation of tumors by preventing the formation of carcinogens, helping the liver to detoxify and protecting DNA by producing enzymes that speed carcinogen removal and enhance DNA repair activity. Green tea also inhibits tumor promotion by inhibiting abnormal cell growth, slowing the production of hydrogen peroxide and other reactive free radicals and enhancing the immune system.

Green tea polyphenols increase detoxification enzymes, including cytochrome P450, glutathione peroxidase, glutathione reductase, glutathione transferase enzyme, etalase and quinone reductase. These detoxifying enzymes are vitally important to our ability to cope with a diversity of stresses, including the ever-expanding levels of toxins to which we are exposed.

EGCG inhibits u-PA, one the hydrolases implicated in tumor growth. EGCG directly suppresses the activity of matrix metalloproteinase (MMP-2 and MMP-9, both isomers of MMP), two of the protease enzymes frequently overexpressed in cancer and angiogenesis (the formation of new blood vessels essential to cancer growth) and used by tumors to facilitate their spread (Sazuka, et al.). EGCG has also been shown to have anticancer effects in both in vitro and in vivo studies (Boik).

The National Cancer Institute investigated the effect of green tea polyphenols on the induction of apoptosis (programmed cell death) and the regulation of the cell cycle in human and mouse carcinoma cells. Researchers concluded that green tea offers protection against a wide variety of human and mouse tumor cell lines by causing cell cycle arrest and inducing apoptosis (Mukhtar and Cao).

Another study was conducted by Dorothy Morre, a professor of foods and nutrition at Purdue University, and James Morre, a chemist and pharmacologist at Purdue, who had heard reports of green tea's purported effects and set out to see if they were true. Their study demonstrated that growth of human lung cancer cell line PC-9 was inhibited by green tea polyphenols, specifically EGCG (Okabe). Speaking at a meeting of the American Society for Cell Biology in San Francisco, they said that green tea appears to intercept cell division during the mitotic (M-2) stage of cell growth. "Our research shows that green tea leaves are rich in this anticancer compound, with concentrations high enough to induce anticancer effects in the body," said Dorothy Morre.

They also found that green tea affects an enzyme known as NOX (Mukhtar and Cao). "Normal cells express the NOX enzyme only when they are dividing in response to growth hormone signals," said Dorothy Morre. "In contrast, cancer cells have somehow gained the ability to express NOX activity at all times." This tumor-associated NOX activity is called +NOX. The Morres found EGCG interfered with +NOX but not with normal NOX. "This is one of the first studies to directly link the EGCG in green tea to anticancer activity," said Dorothy Morre. The EGCG limits the activity of breast cancer tumor cells grown in the laboratory, but it does not seem to affect normal, healthy breast cells. (Green tea and black tea both come from the same bush in the camellia family, but black tea has been allowed to ferment, which may interfere with compounds such as EGCG.)

A 1998 study indicated that green tea consumption supports women's breast health in a variety of ways and may be one reason that breast cancer remains low in Japan compared with the United States (Boik; Nakachi).

## 15. LO HAN (CUCURBITACEA FRUIT) (*FRUCTUS MOMORDICAE GROSVENORI*)

Traditionally in China, Lo Han has been used as a lung tonic and for stress relief. This herb is 250 times sweeter than common white sugar yet has no negative effects on the body.

## 16. GINGER (*ZINGIBER OFFICINALIS*)

Because of its ability to influence prostaglandin metabolism, ginger is a potent inhibitor of thromboxane synthesis and of platelet aggregation and inflammation. Ginger also has been shown to significantly reduce serum and hepatic cholesterol levels and to possess potent cardiotonic activity and antioxidant effects. Ginger also possesses remarkable proteolytic activity, making it useful for treating many digestive complaints. Ginger relieves chill, coughs and indigestion and counteracts nausea, dizziness, diarrhea, abdominal pain and arthritis. Ginger promotes the secretion of saliva and gastric juices as well as bile. Ginger's effect on circulation is as a gentle, diffusive stimulant; it also has a mild relaxing effect on the circulatory system.

New research has shown that about six compounds (especially [10]shogaol) appear to be important in providing ginger's antiemetic activity (Kawai). The activity of ginger is due to its volatile oil that contains the sesquiterpenes zingiberene and bisabolene and pungent gingerols. Ginger contains curcumin (like tumeric) in addition to the phenolic compounds gingerols and diarylheptanoids, which are high in antioxidants.

# Adaptogens and Cancer Inhibition

Cancer research reveals that herbal adaptogens can play a pivotal role in cancer prevention either by inhibiting carcinogenesis or by stabilizing or reversing premalignant conditions. Adaptogens are also important during active cancer. These herbs can assist the body in coping with the disease while increasing the body's ability to withstand many negative effects of conventional cancer therapies—surgery, chemotherapy and radiation therapies.

Administering adaptogenic plants—including Rhodiola, Schizandra, Resihi, *Curcuma longa* and Eleutherococcus—to cancer patients has shown consistently positive results. There is enough evidence, based on years of research, to conclude that adaptogenic plants, when used regularly, can effectively prevent the development and reoccurrence of cancer, suppress metastases and decrease adverse side effects of conventional cytotoxic therapies. It should be noted, however, that herbal adaptogens tend to be diverse in their actions and require time to invoke their therapeutic effects.

Adaptogens inhibit cancer by enhancing defense systems in a multitude of ways (Fotsis; Herschman; Joshi; Sasaki; Sheng; Subbaramaiah), some of which include:

1. Inhibition of genetic damage by reducing the effects of selective oxygen species (SOS) acting as harmful antioxidants (note: antioxidants can have both harmful and beneficial effects).

2. Stimulation of DNA repair mechanisms in cells able to be repaired or induction of apoptosis (programmed cell death) in cells too damaged to

be repaired, which otherwise could cause oxidative damage such as lipid peroxidation.

3. Increasing the utilization of oxygen and fuel with fewer negative waste by-products such as lactic acid.

4. Assisting in the body's ability to manage stress, therefore increasing vitality.

5. Angiogenesis inhibition, whose mechanisms include the following:

   a. Suppression of beta fibroblast growth factor (bFGF).

   b. Suppression of vascular endothelial growth factor (VEGF).

   c. Inhibition of urokinase-type plasminogen activator (uPA), which contributes to the degradation of the vascular basement membrane and extracellular matrix. According to the results of a prospective 14-center trial, presented by Dr. Anita Prech of Technical University in Munich, Germany, at the 91st annual meeting of the American Association for Cancer Research, women with node-negative breast cancer who have low levels of uPA and plasminogen activator inhibitor type 1 (PAI-l) do not need chemotherapy after surgery (Pennell). (The researchers studied 684 women with node-negative disease between June 1993 and January 1999.)

   d. Inhibition of protein kinase C (PKC).

   e. Inhibition of cyclooxygenase (COX-2). C0X-2 is not detectable in most normal tissues; it is induced by phorbol esters, cytokines and growth factors, including TGF-beta and bFGF, and has been associated with carcinogenesis. COX-2, but not COX-l, was found to be up-regulated in several human cancers, including colon, gastric, breast, prostate, bladder, lung and squamous cell carcinoma.

The ability of flavonoids to inhibit cancer appears to be similar to many other natural food phytonutrients. They act via the liver and influence its detoxifying enzyme systems to induce phase II detoxification of quinone reductase and inhibit ornithine decarboxylase (ODC), an enzyme involved in cancer synthesis and tumor promotion. Proanthocyanidin and anthocyanidin inhibited all the phases of the lipid peroxidative cascade and the induction initiated by hydrogen peroxide.

Proanthocyanidins have shown antioxidant ability 10 times greater than that of vitamin E.

A recent study using grape seed proanthocyanidin extract (GSPE) in vitro along with Chang liver cells (a cell line commonly used to study cancer) treated with two popular chemotherapeutic agents, adriamycin and cytoxin, found that GSPE is a potential candidate to ameliorate the toxic effects of these cancer drugs. Compared with untreated Chang liver cells, the GSPE-treated cells showed decreased expression of several important cell-cycle-related genes, including p53 and c-myc (Joshi).

Ellagic acid is another important phenolic constituent found in many berries and nuts. Pomegranates are the richest source of ellagic acid, but raspberries, blackberries, elderberries, marionberries, boysenberries and loganberries possess it too. Ellagic acid inhibits cancer formation and is believed to inhibit cancer mutation by latching onto sensitive sites on the DNA that might otherwise be occupied by harmful chemicals. Ellagic acid is particularly effective in the inhibition of lung cancer caused by cigarette smoking. If you don't already consume a variety of berries in your diet, we recommend that you and your loved ones eat them regularly.

# Summary of Benefits of the Hot 16 Adaptogens

1. **Siberian Ginseng (*Eleutherococcus senticosus*)**
   - Helps your body cope with stress.
   - Improves your mental alertness.
   - Helps your body cure itself of colds and infections.
   - Improves your overall health.
   - Lowers your cholesterol and blood pressure.

2. **American and Korean Ginseng (*Panax quinquefolius/ ginseng*)**
   - Helps your body adapt to stress.
   - Normalizes your body functions.
   - Acts as a mild tonic.
   - Enhances your physical and mental performance.
   - Lowers your cholesterol.
   - May inhibit the growth of cancerous tumors.

3. **Pantocrene (extracted from the velvet of Siberian Deer Antler)**
   - Boosts your energy.
   - Builds muscle.
   - Relieves inflammation and can be effective against arthritis.
   - Acts as an aphrodisiac and sexual tonic.

4. **Arctic Root (*Rhodiola rosea*)**
   - Protects your nervous and endocrine systems.
   - Acts as an anticarcinogenic, antimetastic and antimutagenic.

- Protects against altitude sickness.
- Assists your body during time of stress, especially cardiac stress.
- Promotes the regeneration process of your immune system.
- Shortens the recovery time of suppressed white blood cells following chemotherapy or radiation therapy.

## 5. Schizandra (Seed and Fruit)
- Fortifies and strengthens your body.
- Enhances your resistance to disease and stress.
- Increases stamina and improves athletic performance.
- Improves your overall health and vitality.
- Provides antitoxic and antioxidant activity against many toxic chemicals.
- Protects DNA from damage.
- Improves sleep.

## 6. Ashwagandha Root (*Withania somnifera*)
- Increases your stamina and vitality.
- Helps your body fight disease.
- Acts as a sexual rejuvenator for men.
- Relieves symptoms of arthritis.

## 7. Oats (Straw, Grain and Fresh Milky Unripe Seed) (*Avena sativa*)
- Helps against gas and upset stomach.
- Protects against heart disease by reducing cholesterol.
- Is a good source of B vitamins.
- Has a calming effect on your body.
- Nourishes your nervous system.
- Is rich in calcium and magnesium.
- Helps with nervous exhaustion, anxiety, impaired sleep patterns, weakness and poor libido.

## 8. Reishi Mushroom (*Ganoderma lucidum*)
- Enhances your immune system.
- Helps alleviate arthritis discomfort.
- Increases longevity.

- Restores homeostasis.
- Enhances your energy.
- Prevents and combats altitude sickness.

## 9. Cordyceps (*Cordyceps sinesis*)
- Improves physical endurance.
- Fortifies your body against stress.
- Acts as a restorative tonic.
- Enhances immunity.
- Acts as an antiasthmatic.
- Replenishes sperm.
- Acts as a tonic for renal, hepatic, respiratory, nervous and cardio-vascular systems.

## 10. Licorice (*Glycyrrhiza glabra*)
- Reduces the pain of ulcers.
- Relieves menopausal symptoms.
- Breaks up congestion due to colds.
- Soothes sore, hoarse throats.
- Reduces pain and stiffness.
- Retards the growth of certain cancers.
- Helps in the treatment of hepatitis B.
- Has a regulating effect on certain hormones.
- Acts as a potent antitoxin, lowering the toxicity of many sub-stances such as strychnine, histamine, arsenate, snake venom, diphtheria and tetanus.
- Acts as an anti-inflammatory.
- Improves the tone of your digestive system.

## 11. Elderberry (*Sambuccua canadensis nigra*)
- Relieves symptoms of coughs and colds.
- Acts as a potent free-radical scavenger, thus reducing oxidative stress.
- Enhances immunity.
- Acts as an antiviral force.
- Provides cardiovascular protection.
- Reduces stress.

## 12. Hawthorn (Leaves, Blossoms and Berries) (*Crataegus oxyacantha*)
- Enhances cardiovascular health.
- Improves circulation.
- Helps treat heart failure and angina.
- Lowers blood pressure.

## 13. Grape Seed and Skin Extract (*Vitis vinifera*)
- Acts as a potent antioxidant—it's 20 to 50 times more powerful than vitamins C and E.
- Protects against hardening of the arteries.
- Acts as an anti-inflammatory.
- Fights cancer.
- Builds collagen.
- Inhibits natural COX-2.

## 14. Green Tea (*Camellia sinensis*)
- Controls free radicals.
- Reduces the risk of cancer.
- Helps detoxify the liver and protects DNA.
- Helps prevent heart disease.

## 15. Lo Han (Cucurbitaceae fruit) (*Fructus momordicae grosvenori*)
- Acts as a lung tonic.
- Relieves stress.
- Is a potent sweetener (250 times sweeter than white sugar with no negative effects).

## 16. Ginger (*Zingiber officinalis*)
- Influences prostaglandin metabolism.
- Inhibits clumping together of platelets.
- Acts as an anti-inflammatory.
- Reduces cholesterol.
- Acts as an antioxidant and tonic for the cardiovascular system.
- Aids digestion.
- Acts as an antinausea agent.

# References

Arase, Y., et al., 1997. "The long-term efficacy of glycyrrhizin in chronic hepatitis patients." *Cancer* 79 (8): l494–1500.

Boik, J. *Natural Compounds in Cancer Therapy.* Princeton, Minn.: Oregon Medical Press, 2001, pp. 260–63, 307–309.

Cheng, H. H., et al., 1988. "The immunomodulatory effects of ganoderma polysaccharides and its mechanisms." *Journal of Chinese Oncology Society* 4: 13.

*Chinese Herbal Medicine Materia Medica,* translated by D. Bensky and A. Gamble, rev. ed., 1993. Seattle: Eastland Press, pp. 336–73.

Dannenberg, A. J., quoted in Harris, R. E., et al., 2000. "Chemoprevention of breast cancer in rats by celecoxib, a cyclooxygenase-2 inhibitor." *Cancer Research* 60: 2101–03. (Source: Medscape, Sept. 6, 2000.)

Devi, P. U., 1996. "*Withania somnifera* (Ashwagandha): potential plant source of a promising drug for cancer chemotherapy and adiosensitization." *Indian Journal of Experimental Biology* 34 (10): 927–32.

*Donald Brown's Quarterly Review of Natural Medicine,* Summer 1995.

Duke, J. *Ginseng: A Concise Handbook.* Algonac, Mich.: Reference Publications, 1989.

Ellingwood, Finley. *American Materia Medica, Therapeutics.* Cincinnati, Ohio: Eclectic Medical Publications, 1919, pp. 204–06.

Foster, S. *Siberian Ginseng.* American Botanical Council, Botanical Series, no. 302.

Fotsis, T., et al., 1997. "Flavonoids, dietary-derived inhibitors of cell proliferation and in vitro angiogenesis." *Cancer Research* 57: 2916–21.

Frances, D. *Medicines from the Earth 2001, Plants as Teachers: Nymphace adorara.* Brevard, N.C.: Gaia Herbal Research Institute, 2001.

Fulder, S. *The Root of Being: Ginseng and the Pharmacology of Harmony.* London: Hutchinson, 1980.

_____, 1980. "The drug that builds Russians." *New Scientist* 87: 576–90.

Ganasoundari, A., et al., 1997. "Modification of bone marrow radiosensitivity by medical plant extracts." *British Journal of Radiology* 70(834): 599–602.

Grandhi, A., et al., 1994. "A comparative pharmacological investigation of ashwagandha and ginseng."*Journal of Ethnopharmacology* 44 (131): 11994.

Harris, R. E., et al., 2000. "Chemoprevention of breast cancer in rats by celecoxib, a cyclooxygenase-2 inhibitor." *Cancer Research* 60: 2101–03.

Herschman, H. R., 1994. "Regulation of prostaglandin synthase-1 and prostaglandin synthase-2. *Cancer Metastasis Review* 13: 241–56.

Ho, C-T., et al. *Food Phytochemicals for Cancer Prevention II: Teas, Spices and Herbs.* Washington, D.C.: American Chemical Society, 1994, pp. 342–54

Hobbs, C. *Medical Mushrooms.* Loveland, Colo.: Botanica Press, 1995.

Huang, K. C. *The Pharmacology of Chinese Herbs.* Boca Raton, Fla.: RC Press, 1999, pp. 118–20, 263–64, 364–69.

Jianzhe, Y., et al. *Icons of Medicinal Fengi from China.* Beijing: Science Press, 1987.

Joshi, S. S., et al., 2000. "Chemopreventive effects of grape seed proanthocyanidin extract on Chang liver cells." *Toxicology* 155: 83–90.

Kawai, T., et al., 1994. "Anti-emetic principles of Mognolia obovato bark and Zingiber off. Rhizome." *Planta Medica* 60: 17.

Kelly, Gregory S., 1999. "Nutritional and botanical interventions to assist with the adaptation to stress." *Alternative Medicine Review* 4: 249–60.

Kuo, Y. C., et al., 1994. "Cordyceps sinensis as an immunomodulatory agent." *Cancer Investigation* 12 (6): 611.

Lien, E., and Li, W. *Anticancer Chinese Drugs.* Taiwan: Oriental Healing Arts Institute, 1985, p. 116.

Lucci, L. R., 2000. "Selected herbals and human exercise performance." *American Journal of Clinical Nutrition* 72: 6245–6365.

Mills, S., and Bone, K. "Ginseng," in *Principles and Practice of Phytotherapy.* London: Livingston Churchill, 2000, pp. 418–32.

Mukhtar, H., and Cao, Y., 2000. "Green tea experiments in lab clinic yield mixed results." *Journal of the National Cancer Institutes* 92 (13): 1038–09.

Nakachi, K., et al., 1998. "Influence of drinking green tea on breast cancer malignancy among Japanese patients." *Japanese Journal of Cancer Research* 89: 254–61.

Odintsev, S. N., et al., 1992. "The enhancement of the efficacy of Adriamycin by using hepatoprotectors of plant origin in metastases of Ehrlich's adenocarcinoma to the liver in mice." Vopr. Onkol. 38: 1217–22.

Ohmori, T., et al., 1989. "Antitumor activity of protein-bound polysaccharide from cordyceps in mice." *Japanese Journal of Experimental Medicine* 59 (4): 157–61.

Okabe, S., et al., 1997. "Mechanism of growth inhibition of human lung cancer cell line, PC-9, by tea polyphenols." *Japanese Journal of Cancer Research* 88 (7): 639–43.

Pennell, M. M., 2000. "Tumor factor assay guides treatment of women with node-negative breast cancer." *Reuters Health,* Apr. 10.

Porter, S., 2000. Unpublished study conducted in1999. HerbalGram 50: 56.

Sasaki, E., et al., 1998. "Induction of cyclooxygenase-2 in rat gastric epithelial cell line by epiregulin and basic fibroblast growth factor." *Journal of Clinical Gastroenterology* 27 (supplement 1): S21–S27.

Sazuka, M., et al., 1997. "Inhibition of collagenases from mouse lung carcinoma cells by green tea catechins." *Bioscience, Biotechnology, Biochemistry* 9: 1504–06.

Sheng, H., et al., 1997. "Cyclooxygenase-2 induction and transforming growth factor-growth inhibition in rat intestinal epithelial cells." *Cell Growth Differentiation* 8: 463–72.

Sinclair, S., et al., 1998. "Chinese herbs: a clinical review of astragalus, ligustrum and schizandra." *Alternative Medical Review* 3 (5): 338–44.

Stancheva, S. L., and Mosharrof, A., 1987. "Effect of the extract of *Rhodiola rosea L.* on the content of the brain biogenic monamines." *Medical Physiology* 40: 85–87.

Subbaramaiah, K., et al., 1996. "Transcription of cyclooxygenase-2 is enhanced in transformed mammary epithelial cells." *Cancer Research* 56, 4424–29.

Wahlstrom, M., 1987. "Adaptogens." *Herbal Healthline* (3): 13.

Yaremenko, K. V., and Pashinski, V. G., 1986. "Preparations of natural origin as remedies for prophylactic oncology." *New Medical Preparations from Plants of Siberia and the Far East,* pp. 171–72.

Zhou, D. H., and Lin, L. Z., 1995. *Journal of Chinese Traditional Medicine* 15: 476.

Zhou, J., and G. Liu. *Recent Advances in Chinese Medicine.* Beijing: Science Press, 1991, pp. 133–41.

# Index

# About the Authors

**Earl Mindell, R.Ph., Ph.D.**

Earl Mindell, R.Ph., Ph.D. is a professor of nutrition at Pacific Western University. In addition to writing several hundred articles on the subject of alternative health, Dr. Mindell has written more than thirty books and booklets, including the bestselling *Earl Mindell's Vitamin Bible* and *Earl Mindell's Herb Bible.* Dr. Mindell received his pharmacy degree from North Dakota State University and his doctorate in nutrition from Pacific Western University.

**Donald R. Yance, Jr., M.H., C.N., A.H.G., S.F.O.**

Donald Yance, Jr. is a practicing clinical master herbalist and certified nutritionist specializing in the use of nutritional and herbal approaches to cancer, AIDS, heart disease and other chronic health conditions, as complementary and/or primary therapies and in the prevention of disease. Mr. Yance is the author of *Herbal Medicine, Healing and Cancer.* He also writes and reviews articles for several nutritional and herbal journals, including *Alternative Medicine Journal, Prevention Magazine, Self Magazine* and *Vegetarian Times,* and he contributes a bimonthly article, "An Herbal Case History," to *Total Health.*